Mediterranean Quick Delights

50 Easy-to-Make Recipes for Quick & Delicious Mediterranean Meals

Ken Bartiromo

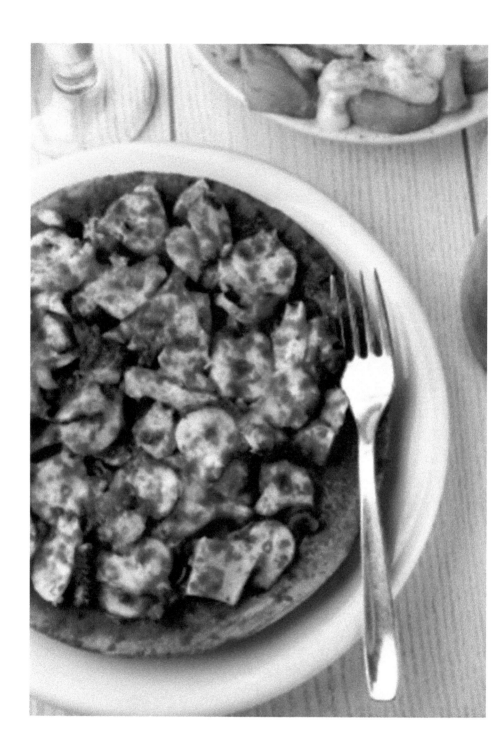

© Copyright 2021 - All rights reserved.

The content contained within this book may not be reproduced, duplicated or transmitted without direct written permission from the author or the publisher.
Under no circumstances will any blame or legal responsibility be held against the publisher, or author, for any damages, reparation, or monetary loss due to the information contained within this book. Either directly or indirectly.

Legal Notice:
This book is copyright protected. This book is only for personal use. You cannot amend, distribute, sell, use, quote or paraphrase any part, or the content within this book, without the consent of the author or publisher.

Disclaimer Notice:
Please note the information contained within this document is for educational and entertainment purposes only. All effort has been executed to present accurate, up to date, and reliable, complete information. No warranties of any kind are declared or implied. Readers acknowledge that the author is not engaging in the rendering of legal, financial, medical or professional advice. The content within this book has been derived from various sources. Please consult a licensed professional before attempting any techniques outlined in this book.
By reading this document, the reader agrees that under no circumstances is the author responsible for any losses, direct or indirect, which are incurred as a result of the use of information contained within this document, including, but not limited to, — errors, omissions, or inaccuracies.

Table of Contents

Oven-grilled Oyster Mushroom Meal

Difficulty Level: 2/5

Preparation time: 10 minutes

Cooking time: 15 minutes

Servings: 4

Ingredients:

20-oz. oyster mushrooms

2-tbsp extra-virgin olive oil

Salt and freshly ground pepper

2-tsp parsley, minced

Directions:

Preheat your oven to 420 °F.

Line a 5" x 9" baking sheet with foil, and spray the surfaces with non-stick grease. Set aside.

Meanwhile, prepare the mushrooms by separating and discarding their stems. By using a damp towel or a mushroom brush, clean their top surfaces.

Spray or brush the mushrooms with the olive oil. Place and arrange the mushrooms in a baking sheet. Grill for 5 minutes. (Grill for an additional 4 minutes for thicker mushrooms.

Take out the sheet, and place the grilled mushrooms in a serving platter. Sprinkle over with salt and freshly ground pepper. Top them with parsley, and serve immediately.

Nutrition:

Calories: 107

Total Fats: 7.3g

Fiber: 3.3g

Carbohydrates: 8.7g

Protein: 4.7g

Grilled Burgers with Mushrooms

Difficulty Level: 2/5

Preparation time: 10 minutes

Cooking time: 10 minutes

Servings: 4

Ingredients:

2 Bibb lettuce, halved

4 slices red onion

4 slices tomato

4 whole wheat buns, toasted

2 tbsp olive oil

¼ tsp cayenne pepper, optional

1 garlic clove, minced

1 tbsp sugar

½ cup water

1/3 cup balsamic vinegar

4 large Portobello mushroom caps, around 5-inches in diameter

Directions:

Remove stems from mushrooms and clean with a damp cloth. Transfer into a baking dish with gill-side up.

In a bowl, mix thoroughly olive oil, cayenne pepper, garlic, sugar, water and vinegar. Pour over mushrooms and marinate mushrooms in the ref for at least an hour.

Once the one hour is nearly up, preheat grill to medium high fire and grease grill grate.

Grill mushrooms for five minutes per side or until tender. Baste mushrooms with marinade so it doesn't dry up.

To assemble, place ½ of bread bun on a plate, top with a slice of onion, mushroom, tomato and one lettuce leaf. Cover with the other top half of the bun. Repeat process with remaining ingredients, serve and enjoy.

Nutrition:

Calories: 244.1

Fiber: 9.3g

Carbohydrates: 32g

Protein: 8.1g

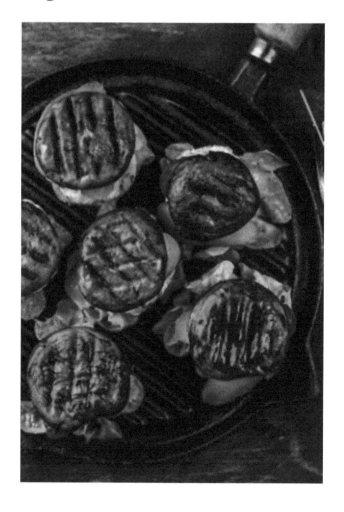

Mediterranean Baba Ghanoush

Difficulty Level: 3/5

Preparation time: 5 minutes

Cooking time: 25 minutes

Servings: 4

Ingredients:

1 bulb garlic

1 red bell pepper, halved and seeded

1 tbsp chopped fresh basil

1 tbsp olive oil

1 tsp black pepper

2 eggplants, sliced lengthwise

2 rounds of flatbread or pita

Juice of 1 lemon

Directions:

Grease grill grate with cooking spray and preheat grill to medium high.

Slice tops of garlic bulb and wrap in foil. Place in the cooler portion of the grill and roast for at least 20 minutes.

Place bell pepper and eggplant slices on the hottest part of grill.

Grill for at least two to three minutes each side.

Once bulbs are done, peel off skins of roasted garlic and place peeled garlic into food processor.

Add olive oil, pepper, basil, lemon juice, grilled red bell pepper and grilled eggplant.

Puree until smooth and transfer into a bowl.

Grill bread at least 30 seconds per side to warm.

Serve bread with the pureed dip and enjoy.

Nutrition:

Calories: 213.6

Fiber: 36.3g

Carbohydrates: 6.3g

Protein: 4.8g

Tasty Crabby Panini

Difficulty Level: 2/5

Preparation time: 10 minutes

Cooking time: 10 minutes

Servings: 4

Ingredients:

1 tbsp Olive oil

French bread split and sliced diagonally

1 lb. blue crab meat or shrimp or spiny lobster or stone crab

½ cup celery

¼ cup green onion chopped

1 tsp Worcestershire sauce

1 tsp lemon juice

1 tbsp Dijon mustard

½ cup light mayonnaise

Directions:

In a medium bowl mix the following thoroughly: celery, onion, Worcestershire, lemon juice, mustard and mayonnaise. Season with pepper and salt. Then gently add in the almonds and crabs.

Spread olive oil on sliced sides of bread and smear with crab mixture before covering with another bread slice.

Grill sandwich in a Panini press until bread is crisped and ridged.

Nutrition:

Calories: 248

Fiber: 10.9g

Carbohydrates: 12.0g

Protein: 24.5g

Bean and Toasted Pita Salad

Difficulty Level: 2/5

Preparation time: 15 minutes

Cooking time: 10 minutes

Servings: 4

Ingredients:

3 tbsp chopped fresh mint

3 tbsp chopped fresh parsley

1 cup crumbled feta cheese

1 cup sliced romaine lettuce

½ cucumber, peeled and sliced

1 cup diced plum tomatoes

2 cups cooked pinto beans, well drained and slightly warmed

Pepper to taste

3 tbsp extra virgin olive oil

2 tbsp ground toasted cumin seeds

2 tbsp fresh lemon juice

1/8 tsp salt

2 cloves garlic, peeled

2 6-inch whole wheat pita bread, cut or torn into bite-sized pieces

Directions:

In large baking sheet, spread torn pita bread and bake in a preheated 4000F oven for 6 minutes.

With the back of a knife, mash garlic and salt until paste like. Add into a medium bowl.

Whisk in ground cumin and lemon juice. In a steady and slow stream, pour oil as you whisk continuously. Season with pepper.

In a large salad bowl, mix cucumber, tomatoes and beans. Pour in dressing, toss to coat well.

Add mint, parsley, feta, lettuce and toasted pita, toss to mix once again and serve.

Nutrition:

Calories: 427

Carbohydrates: 47.3g

Protein: 17.7g

Fat: 20.4g

Goat Cheese 'n Red Beans Salad

Difficulty Level: 1/5

Preparation time: 15 minutes

Cooking time: 0 minutes

Servings: 4

Ingredients:

2 cans of Red Kidney Beans, drained and rinsed well

Water or vegetable broth to cover beans

1 bunch parsley, chopped

1 1/2 cups red grape tomatoes, halved

3 cloves garlic, minced

3 tablespoons olive oil

3 tablespoons lemon juice

1/2 teaspoon salt

1/2 teaspoon white pepper

6 ounces goat cheese, crumbled

Directions:

In a large bowl, combine beans, parsley, tomatoes and garlic.

Add olive oil, lemon juice, salt and pepper.

Mix well and refrigerate until ready to serve.

Spoon into individual dishes topped with crumbled goat cheese.

Nutrition:

Calories: 385

Carbohydrates: 44.0g

Protein: 22.5g

Fat: 15.0g

Spicy Sweet Red Hummus

Difficulty Level: 1/5

Preparation time: 10 minutes

Cooking time: 0 minutes

Servings: 8

Ingredients:

1 (15 ounce) can garbanzo beans, drained

1 (4 ounce) jar roasted red peppers

1 1/2 tablespoons tahini

1 clove garlic, minced

1 tablespoon chopped fresh parsley

1/2 teaspoon cayenne pepper

1/2 teaspoon ground cumin

1/4 teaspoon salt

3 tablespoons lemon juice

Directions:

In a blender, add all ingredients and process until smooth and creamy.

Adjust seasoning to taste if needed.

Can be stored in an airtight container for up to 5 days.

Nutrition:

Calories: 64

Carbohydrates: 9.6g

Protein: 2.5g

Fat: 2.2g

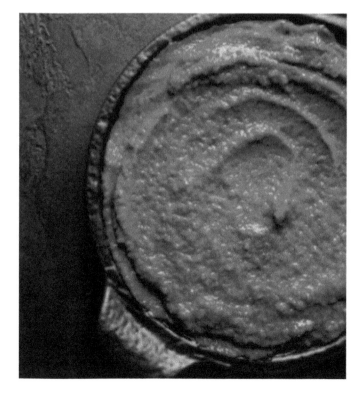

Dill Relish on White Sea Bass

Difficulty Level: 2/5

Preparation time: 15 minutes

Cooking time: 12 minutes

Servings: 4

Ingredients:

1 ½ tbsp chopped white onion

1 ½ tsp chopped fresh dill

1 lemon, quartered

1 tsp Dijon mustard

1 tsp lemon juice

1 tsp pickled baby capers, drained

4 pieces of 4-oz white sea bass fillets

Directions:

Preheat oven to 375oF.

Mix lemon juice, mustard, dill, capers and onions in a small bowl.

Prepare four aluminum foil squares and place 1 fillet per foil.

Squeeze a lemon wedge per fish.

Evenly divide into 4 the dill spread and drizzle over fillet.

Close the foil over the fish securely and pop in the oven.

Bake for 10 to 12 minutes or until fish is cooked through.

Remove from foil and transfer to a serving platter, serve and enjoy.

Nutrition:

Calories: 115

Carbohydrates: 12g

Protein: 7g

Fat: 1g

Vegetable Lover's Chicken Soup

Difficulty Level: 2/5

Preparation time: 10 minutes

Cooking time: 20 minutes

Servings: 4

Ingredients:

1 ½ cups baby spinach

2 tbsp orzo (tiny pasta)

¼ cup dry white wine

1 14oz low sodium chicken broth

2 plum tomatoes, chopped

1/8 tsp salt

½ tsp Italian seasoning

1 large shallot, chopped

1 small zucchini, diced

8-oz chicken tenders

1 tbsp extra virgin olive oil

Directions:

In a large saucepan, heat oil over medium heat and add the chicken. Stir occasionally for 8 minutes until browned. Transfer in a plate. Set aside.

In the same saucepan, add the zucchini, Italian seasoning, shallot and salt and stir often until the vegetables are softened, around 4 minutes.

Add the tomatoes, wine, broth and orzo and increase the heat to high to bring the mixture to boil. Reduce the heat and simmer.

Add the cooked chicken and stir in the spinach last.

Serve hot.

Nutrition:

Calories: 207

Carbohydrates: 14.8g

Protein: 12.2g

Fat: 11.4g

Mustard Chops with Apricot-basil Relish

Difficulty Level: 2/5

Preparation time: 18 minutes

Cooking time: 12 minutes

Servings: 4

Ingredients:

¼ cup basil, finely shredded

¼ cup olive oil

½ cup mustard

¾ lb. fresh apricots, stone removed, and fruit diced

1 shallot, diced small

1 tsp ground cardamom

3 tbsp raspberry vinegar

4 pork chops

Pepper and salt

Directions:

Make sure that pork chops are defrosted well. Season with pepper and salt. Slather both sides of each pork chop with mustard. Preheat grill to medium-high fire.

In a medium bowl, mix cardamom, olive oil, vinegar, basil, shallot, and apricots. Toss to combine and season with pepper and salt, mixing once again.

Grill chops for 5 to 6 minutes per side. As you flip, baste with mustard.

Serve pork chops with the Apricot-Basil relish and enjoy.

Nutrition:

Calories: 486.5

Carbohydrates: 7.3g

Protein: 42.1g

Fat: 32.1g

Seafood and Veggie Pasta

Difficulty Level: 3/5

Preparation time: 10 minutes

Cooking time: 20 minutes

Servings: 4

Ingredients:

¼ tsp pepper

¼ tsp salt

1 lb raw shelled shrimp

1 lemon, cut into wedges

1 tbsp butter

1 tbsp olive oil

2 5-oz cans chopped clams, drained (reserve 2 tbsp clam juice)

2 tbsp dry white wine

4 cloves garlic, minced

4 cups zucchini, spiraled (use a veggie spiralizer)

4 tbsp Parmesan Cheese

Chopped fresh parsley to garnish

Directions:

Ready the zucchini and spiralize with a veggie spiralizer. Arrange 1 cup of zucchini noodle per bowl. Total of 4 bowls.

On medium fire, place a large nonstick saucepan and heat oil and butter.

For a minute, sauté garlic. Add shrimp and cook for 3 minutes until opaque or cooked.

Add white wine, reserved clam juice and clams. Bring to a simmer and continue simmering for 2 minutes or until half of liquid has evaporated. Stir constantly.

Season with pepper and salt. And if needed add more to taste.

Remove from fire and evenly distribute seafood sauce to 4 bowls.

Top with a tablespoonful of Parmesan cheese per bowl, serve and enjoy.

Nutrition:

Calories: 324.9

Carbohydrates: 12g

Protein: 43.8g

Fat: 11.3g

Creamy Alfredo Fettuccine

Difficulty Level: 2/5

Preparation time: 5 minutes

Cooking time: 25 minutes

Servings: 4

Ingredients:

Grated parmesan cheese

½ cup freshly grated parmesan cheese

1/8 tsp freshly ground black pepper

½ tsp salt

1 cup whipping cream

 2 tbsp butter

8 oz dried fettuccine, cooked and drained

Directions:

On medium high fire, place a big fry pan and heat butter.

Add pepper, salt and cream and gently boil for three to five minutes.

Once thickened, turn off fire and quickly stir in ½ cup of parmesan cheese. Toss in pasta, mix well.

Top with another batch of parmesan cheese and serve.

Nutrition:

Calories: 202

Carbohydrates: 21.1g

Protein: 7.9g

Fat: 10.2g

Tasty Lasagna Rolls

Difficulty Level: 2/5

Preparation time: 10 minutes

Cooking time: 20 minutes

Servings: 6

Ingredients:

¼ tsp crushed red pepper

¼ tsp salt

½ cup shredded mozzarella cheese

½ cups parmesan cheese, shredded

1 14-oz package tofu, cubed

1 25-oz can of low-sodium marinara sauce

1 tbsp extra virgin olive oil

12 whole wheat lasagna noodles

2 tbsp Kalamata olives, chopped

3 cloves minced garlic

3 cups spinach, chopped

Directions:

Put enough water on a large pot and cook the lasagna noodles according to package instructions. Drain, rinse and set aside until ready to use.

In a large skillet, sauté garlic over medium heat for 20 seconds. Add the tofu and spinach and cook until the spinach wilts. Transfer this mixture in a bowl and add parmesan olives, salt, red pepper and 2/3 cup of the marinara sauce.

In a pan, spread a cup of marinara sauce on the bottom. To make the rolls, place noodle on a surface and spread ¼ cup of the tofu filling. Roll up and place it on the pan with the marinara sauce. Do this procedure until all lasagna noodles are rolled.

Place the pan over high heat and bring to a simmer. Reduce the heat to medium and let it cook for three more minutes. Sprinkle mozzarella cheese and let the cheese melt for two minutes. Serve hot.

Nutrition:

Calories: 304

Carbohydrates: 39.2g

Protein: 23g

Fat: 19.2g

Tortellini Salad with Broccoli

Difficulty Level: 2/5

Preparation time: 10 minutes

Cooking time: 20 minutes

Servings: 12

Ingredients:

1 red onion, chopped finely

1 cup sunflower seeds

1 cup raisins

3 heads fresh broccoli, cut into florets

2 tsp cider vinegar

½ cup white sugar

½ cup mayonnaise

20-oz fresh cheese filled tortellini

Directions:

In a large pot of boiling water, cook tortellini according to manufacturer's instructions. Drain and rinse with cold water and set aside.

Whisk vinegar, sugar and mayonnaise to create your salad dressing.

Mix together in a large bowl red onion, sunflower seeds, raisins, tortellini and broccoli. Pour dressing and toss to coat.

Serve and enjoy.

Nutrition:

Calories: 272

Carbohydrates: 38.7g

Protein: 5.0g

Fat: 8.1g

Simple Penne Anti-Pasto

Difficulty Level: 2/5

Preparation time: 15 minutes

Cooking time: 15 minutes

Servings: 4

Ingredients:

¼ cup pine nuts, toasted

½ cup grated Parmigiano-Reggiano cheese, divided

8oz penne pasta, cooked and drained

1 6oz jar drained, sliced, marinated and quartered artichoke hearts

1 7 oz jar drained and chopped sun-dried tomato halves packed in oil

3 oz chopped prosciutto

1/3 cup pesto

½ cup pitted and chopped Kalamata olives

1 medium red bell pepper

Directions:

Slice bell pepper, discard membranes, seeds and stem. On a foiled lined baking sheet, place bell pepper halves, press down by hand and broil in oven for eight minutes. Remove from oven, put in a sealed bag for 5 minutes before peeling and chopping.

Place chopped bell pepper in a bowl and mix in artichokes, tomatoes, prosciutto, pesto and olives.

Toss in ¼ cup cheese and pasta. Transfer to a serving dish and garnish with ¼ cup cheese and pine nuts. Serve and enjoy!

Nutrition:

Calories: 606

Carbohydrates: 70.3g

Protein: 27.2g

Fat: 27.6g

Butternut Squash Hummus

Difficulty Level: 2/5

Preparation time: 15 minutes

Cooking time: 15 minutes

Servings: 8

Ingredients:

2 pounds butternut squash, seeded and peeled

1 tablespoon olive oil

¼ cup tahini

2 tablespoons lemon juice

2 cloves of garlic, minced

Salt and pepper to taste

Directions:

Heat the oven to 3000F.

Coat the butternut squash with olive oil.

Place in a baking dish and bake for 15 minutes in the oven.

Once the squash is cooked, place in a food processor together with the rest of the ingredients.

Pulse until smooth.

Place in individual containers.

Put a label and store in the fridge.

Allow to warm at room temperature before heating in the microwave oven.

Serve with carrots or celery sticks.

Nutrition:

Calories: 115

Carbohydrates: 15.8g

Protein: 2.5g

Fat: 5.8g

Fiber: 6.7g

Chicken in Tomato-Balsamic Pan Sauce

Difficulty Level: 2/5

Preparation time: 10 minutes

Cooking time: 20 minutes

Servings: 4

Ingredients:

2 (8 oz. or 226.7 g each) boneless chicken breasts, skinless

½ tsp. salt

½ tsp. ground pepper

3 tbsps. extra-virgin olive oil

½ c. halved cherry tomatoes

2 tbsps. sliced shallot

¼ c. balsamic vinegar

1 tbsp. minced garlic

1 tbsp. toasted fennel seeds, crushed

1 tbsp. butter

Directions:

Slice the chicken breasts into 4 pieces and beat them with a mallet till it reaches a thickness of a ¼ inch. Use ¼ teaspoons of pepper and salt to coat the chicken.

Heat two tablespoons of oil in a skillet and keep the heat to a medium. Cook the chicken breasts for three minutes on each side. Transfer it to a serving plate and cover it with foil to keep it warm.

Add one tablespoon oil, shallot, and tomatoes in a pan and cook till it softens. Add vinegar and boil the mix till the vinegar gets reduced by half. Put fennel seeds, garlic, salt, and pepper and cook for about four minutes.

Remove it from the heat and stir it with butter.

Pour this sauce over chicken and serve.

Nutrition:

Calories 294

Fat 17 g

Sat. fat 4 g

Fiber 2 g

Carbohydrates 10 g

Sugar 3 g

Protein 25 g

Brown Rice, Feta, Fresh Pea, and Mint Salad

Difficulty Level: 2/5

Preparation time: 5 minutes

Cooking time: 25 minutes

Servings: 4

Ingredients:

2 c. brown rice

3 c. water

Salt

5 oz. or 141.7 g crumbled feta cheese

2 c. cooked peas

½ c. chopped mint, fresh

2 tbsps. olive oil

Salt and pepper

Directions:

Place the brown rice, water, and salt into a saucepan over medium heat, cover, and bring to boiling point.

Turn the lower heat and allow it to cook until the water has dissolved and the rice is soft but chewy. Leave to cool completely

Add the feta, peas, mint, olive oil, salt, and pepper to a salad bowl with the cooled rice and toss to combine

Serve and enjoy!

Nutrition:

Calories 613

Fat 18.2 g

Sat. fat 7 g

Fiber 12 g

Carbohydrates 45 g

Sugars 9.8 g

Protein 21 g

Sodium 302 mg

Whole Grain Pita Bread Stuffed with Olives and Chickpeas

Difficulty Level: 2/5

Preparation time: 10 minutes

Cooking time: 20 minutes

Servings: 2

Ingredients:

2 wholegrain pita pockets

2 tbsps. olive oil

2 garlic cloves, chopped

1 onion, chopped

½ tsp. cumin

10 black olives, chopped

2 c. cooked chickpeas

Salt and pepper

Directions:

Slice open the pita pockets and set aside

Adjust your heat to medium and set a pan in place. Add in the olive oil and heat.

Add the garlic, onion, and cumin to the hot pan and stir as the onions soften and the cumin is fragrant

Add the olives, chickpeas, salt, and pepper and toss everything together until the chickpeas become golden

Set the pan from heat and use your wooden spoon to roughly mash the chickpeas so that some are intact and some are crushed

Heat your pita pockets in the microwave, in the oven, or on a clean pan on the stove

Fill them with your chickpea mixture and enjoy!

Nutrition:

Calories 503

Fat 19 g

Sat. fat 8.9 g

Fiber 14 g

Carbohydrates 54 g

Sugars 9 g

Protein 15.7 g

Sodium 276 mg

Seasoned Buttered Chicken

Difficulty Level: 2/5

Preparation time: 10 minutes

Cooking time: 20 minutes

Servings: 4

Ingredients:

½ c. heavy whipping cream

1 tbsp. salt

½ c. bone broth

1 tbsp. pepper

4 tbsps. butter

4 chicken breast halves

Directions:

Place cooking pan on your oven over medium heat and add in one tablespoon of butter. Once the butter is warm and melted, place the chicken in and cook for five minutes on either side. At the end of this time, the chicken should be cooked through and golden; if it is, go ahead and place it on a plate.

Next, you are going to add the bone broth into the warm pan. Add heavy whipping cream, salt, and pepper. Then, leave the pan alone until your sauce begins to simmer. Allow this process to happen for five minutes to let the sauce thicken up.

Finally, you are going to add the rest of your butter and the chicken back into the pan. Be sure to use a spoon to place the sauce over your chicken and smother it completely. After a few minutes, your dish will be complete and ready to serve!

Nutrition:

Calories 350

Fat 25 g

Sat. fat 13 g

Fiber 10 g

Carbohydrates 17 g

Sugars 2 g

Protein 25 g

Shrimps with Lemon and Pepper

Difficulty Level: 2/5

Preparation time: 15 minutes

Cooking time: 10 minutes

Servings: 4

Ingredients:

40 deveined shrimps, peeled

6 minced garlic cloves

Salt and black pepper

3 tbsps. olive oil

¼ tsp. sweet paprika

A pinch crushed red pepper flakes

¼ tsp. grated lemon zest

3 tbsps. Sherry or another wine

1½ tbsps. sliced chives

Juice of 1 lemon

Directions:

Adjust your heat to medium-high and set a pan in place.

Add oil and shrimp, sprinkle with pepper and salt and cook for 1 minute

Add paprika, garlic and pepper flakes, stir and cook for 1 minute.

Gently stir in sherry and allow to cook for an extra minute

Take shrimp off the heat, add chives and lemon zest, stir and transfer shrimp to plates.

Add lemon juice all over and serve

Nutrition:

Calories 140

Fat 1 g

Sat. fat 0.3 g

Fiber 0 g

Carbohydrates 1 g

Sugars 0 g

Protein 18 g

Sodium 200 mg

Breaded and Spiced Halibut

Difficulty Level: 2/5

Preparation time: 5 minutes

Cooking time: 25 minutes

Servings: 4

Ingredients:

¼ c. chopped fresh chives

¼ c. chopped fresh dill

¼ tsp. ground black pepper

¾ c. panko breadcrumbs

1 tbsp. extra-virgin olive oil

1 tsp. finely grated lemon zest

1 tsp. sea salt

1/3 c. chopped fresh parsley

4 (6 oz. or 170 g. each) halibut fillets

Directions:

In a medium bowl, mix olive oil and the rest ingredients except halibut fillets and breadcrumbs

Place halibut fillets into the mixture and marinate for 30 minutes

Preheat your oven to 400 F/204 C

Set a foil to a baking sheet, grease with cooking spray

Dip the fillets to the breadcrumbs and put to the baking sheet

Cook in the oven for 20 minutes

Serve hot.

Nutrition:

Calories 667

Fat 24.5 g

Sat. fat 6.5 g

Fiber 2 g

Carbohydrates 30.6 g

Sugars 0.9 g

Protein 54.8 g

Sodium 152 mg

Curry Salmon with Mustard

Difficulty Level: 2/5

Preparation time: 10 minutes

Cooking time: 20 minutes

Servings: 4

Ingredients:

¼ tsp. ground red pepper or chili powder

¼ tsp. turmeric, ground

¼ tsp. salt

1 tsp. honey

¼ tsp. garlic powder

2 tsps. whole grain mustard

4 (6 oz. or 170 g. each) salmon fillets

Directions:

In a bowl mix mustard and the rest ingredients except salmon

Preheat the oven to 350 F/176 C

Grease a baking dish with cooking spray.

Place salmon on baking dish with skin side down and spread evenly mustard mixture on top of fillets

Place into the oven and cook for 10-15 minutes or until flaky.

Nutrition:

Calories 324

Fat 18.9 g

Sat. fat 2 g

Fiber 1.3 g

Carbohydrates 2.9 g

Sugars 1 g

Protein 34 g

Sodium 110 mg

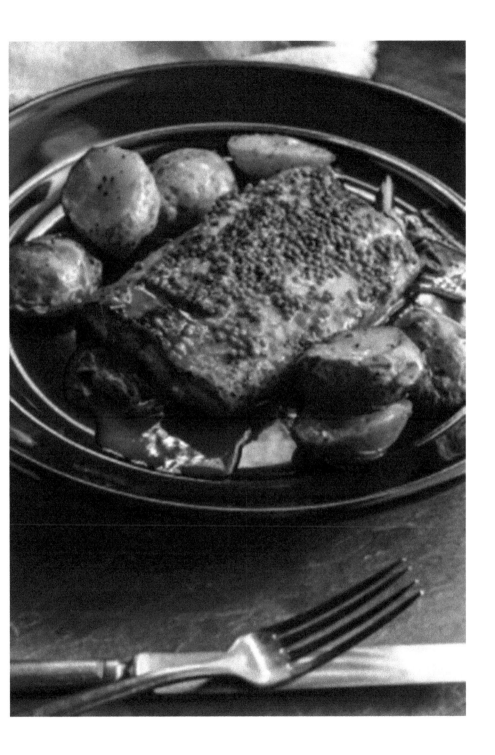

Walnut-Rosemary Crusted Salmon

Difficulty Level: 2/5

Preparation time: 10 minutes

Cooking time: 20 minutes

Servings: 4

Ingredients:

1 lb. or 450 g. frozen skinless salmon fillet

2 tsps. Dijon mustard

1 clove garlic, minced

¼ tsp. lemon zest

½ tsp. honey

½ tsp. kosher salt

1 tsp. freshly chopped rosemary

3 tbsps. panko breadcrumbs

¼ tsp. crushed red pepper

3 tbsps. chopped walnuts

2 tsp. extra-virgin olive oil

Directions:

Preheat the oven to 420 F/215 C and use parchment paper to line a rimmed baking sheet.

In a bowl combine mustard, lemon zest, garlic, lemon juice, honey, rosemary, crushed red pepper, and salt

In another bowl mix walnut, panko, and 1 tsp oil

Place parchments paper on the baking sheet and put the salmon on it

Spread mustard mixture on the fish, and top with the panko mixture.

Spray the rest of olive oil lightly on the salmon.

Bake for about 10 -12 minutes or until the salmon is being separated by a fork

Serve hot

Nutrition:

Calories 222

Fat 12 g

Sat. fat 2 g

Fiber 0.8 g

Carbohydrates 4 g

Sugars 1 g

Protein 24 g

Sodium 256 mg

Quick Tomato Spaghetti

Difficulty Level: 2/5

Preparation time: 10 minutes

Cooking time: 20 minutes

Servings: 4

Ingredients:

8 oz. or 226.7g spaghetti

3 tbsps. olive oil

4 garlic cloves, sliced

1 jalapeno, sliced

2 c. cherry tomatoes

Salt and pepper

1 tsp. balsamic vinegar

½ c. Parmesan, grated

Directions:

Heat a large pot of water on medium flame. Add a pinch of salt and bring to a boil then add the spaghetti.

Allow cooking for 8 minutes.

While the pasta cooks, heat the oil in a skillet and add the garlic and jalapeno. Cook for an extra 1 minute then stir in the tomatoes, pepper, and salt.

Cook for 5-7 minutes until the tomatoes' skins burst.

Add the vinegar and remove off heat.

Drain spaghetti well and mix it with the tomato sauce. Sprinkle with cheese and serve right away.

Nutrition:

Calories 298

Fat 13.5 g

Sat. fat 2.7 g

Fiber 10.5 g

Carbohydrates 36 g

Sugar 8 g

Protein 9.7 g

Sodium 223 mg

Crispy Italian Chicken

Difficulty Level: 2/5

Preparation time: 10 minutes

Cooking time: 20 minutes

Servings: 4

Ingredients:

4 chicken legs

1 tsp. dried basil

1 tsp. dried oregano

Salt and pepper

3 tbsps. olive oil

1 tbsp. balsamic vinegar

Directions:

Season the chicken with salt, pepper, basil, and oregano.

Using a skillet, add oil and heat. Add the chicken in the hot oil.

Let each side cook for 5 minutes until golden then cover the skillet with a lid.

Adjust your heat to medium and cook for 10 minutes on one side then flip the chicken repeatedly, cooking for another 10 minutes until crispy.

Serve the chicken and enjoy.

Nutrition:

Calories: 262

Fat: 13.9 g

Sat. fat: 4 g

Fiber: 0 g

Carbohydrates: 0.3 g

Sugar: 0 g

Protein: 32.6 g

Sodium: 405 mg

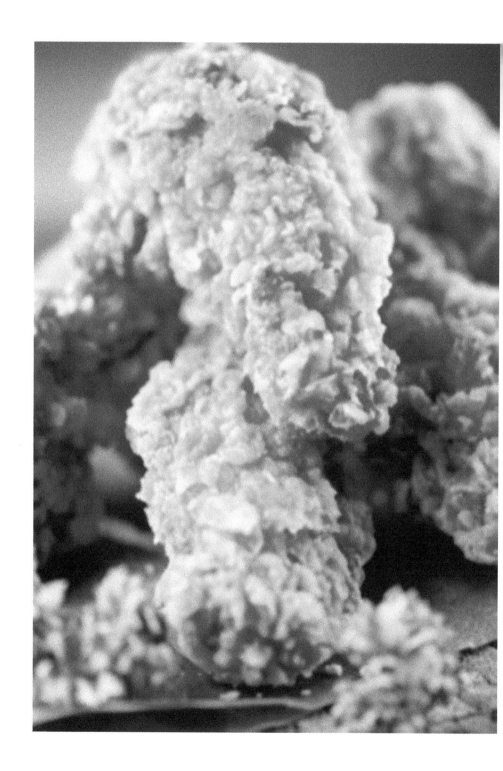

Chili Oregano Baked Cheese

Difficulty Level: 2/5

Preparation time: 5 minutes

Cooking time: 25 minutes

Servings: 4

Ingredients:

8 oz. or 226.7g feta cheese

4 oz. or 113g mozzarella, crumbled

1 sliced chili pepper

1 tsp. dried oregano

2 tbsps. olive oil

Directions:

Place the feta cheese in a small deep-dish baking pan.

Top with the mozzarella then season with pepper slices and oregano.

cover your pan with lid. Cook in the preheated oven at 350 F/176 C for 20 minutes.

Serve the cheese and enjoy it.

Nutrition:

Calories 292

Fat 24.2 g

Sat. fat 7 g

Fiber 2 g

Carbohydrates 5.7 g

Sugar 3 g

Protein 16.2 g

Sodium 287 mg

Sea Bass in a Pocket

Difficulty Level: 2/5

Preparation time: 5 minutes

Cooking time: 25 minutes

Servings: 4

Ingredients:

4 sea bass fillets

4 sliced garlic cloves

1 sliced celery stalk

1 sliced zucchini

1 c. halved cherry tomatoes halved

1 shallot, sliced

1 tsp. dried oregano

Salt and pepper

Directions:

Mix the garlic, celery, zucchini, tomatoes, shallot, and oregano in a bowl. Add salt and pepper to taste.

Take 4 sheets of baking paper and arrange them on your working surface.

Spoon the vegetable mixture in the center of each sheet.

Top with a fish fillet then wrap the paper well so it resembles a pocket.

Place the wrapped fish in a baking tray and cook in the preheated oven at 350 F/176 C for 15 minutes. Serve the fish warm and fresh.

Nutrition:

Calories 149

Fat 2.8 g

Sat. fat 0.7 g

Fiber 0 g

Carbohydrates 5.2 g

Sugar 0 g

Protein 25.2 g

Sodium 87 mg

Tomato Roasted Feta

Difficulty Level: 2/5

Preparation time: 10 minutes

Cooking time: 15 minutes

Servings: 4

Ingredients:

8 oz. or 230 g feta cheese

2 peeled tomatoes, diced

2 garlic cloves, chopped

1 c. tomato juice

1 thyme sprig

1 oregano sprig

Directions:

Mix the tomatoes, garlic, tomato juice, thyme, and oregano in a small deep-dish baking pan.

Place the feta cheese on top and cover with aluminum foil.

Cook in the preheated oven at 350 F/176 C for 10-15 minutes.

Serve hot.

Nutrition:

Calories 173

Fat 12.2 g

Sat fat 6 g

Fiber 2 g

Carbohydrates 7.8 g

Sugars 5 g

Protein 9.2 g

Sodium 934 mg

Shrimp, Avocado and Feta Wrap

Difficulty Level: 2/5

Preparation time: 15 minutes

Cooking time: 10 minutes

Servings: 2

Ingredients:

3 oz. or 85g chopped shrimps, cooked

1 tbsp. lime juice

2 tbsps. crumbled feta cheese

¼ c. diced avocado

1 whole-wheat tortilla

¼ c. diced tomato

1 sliced scallion

Directions:

On a non-stick skillet add shrimps and cook for 5 minutes or until nice pink color

Add feta cheese on the tortilla's one side

Top cheese with the rest ingredients. Add the shrimp on the top so they will be in the middle of the wrap when you roll it.

Add lime juice to give it the tangy zing to the wrap.

Then roll the wrap tightly, but make sure that the ingredients don't fall off.

Then cut the wrap in two halves and serve it.

Nutrition:

Calories 371

Fat 14 g

Sat fat 4 g

Fiber 6 g

Carbohydrates 34 g

Sugars 6 g

Protein 29 g

Sodium 34 mg

Broiled Tilapia Parmesan

Difficulty Level: 2/5

Preparation time: 15 minutes

Cooking time: 15 minutes

Servings: 8

Ingredients:

½ c. Parmesan cheese

¼ c. butter, soft

3 tbsps. mayonnaise

2 tbsps. fresh lemon juice

¼ tsp. dried basil

¼ tsp. ground black pepper

1/8 tsp. onion powder

1/8 tsp. celery salt

2 lbs. or 900 g Tilapia fillets

Directions:

Preheat the grill on your oven. Cover a drip tray or grill pan with aluminum foil.

Combine parmesan, butter, mayonnaise, and lemon juice in a small bowl. Apply a seasoning of onion powder, pepper, dried basil, and celery salt mix well and set aside.

Set the fillets in a single layer on the prepared dish. Grill a few centimeters from the heat for 2 to 3 minutes, turn the fillets and grill for a few minutes.

Remove from oven and cover with Parmesan cheese mixture on top.

Grill for another 2 minutes or until the garnish is golden brown and fish flakes easily with a fork. Be careful not to overcook the fish.

Serve and enjoy!

Nutrition:

Calories 224

Fat 12.8 g

Sat fat 3 g

Fiber 0.2 g

Carbohydrates 0.8 g

Sugars 0 g

Protein 25.4 g

Italian Herb Grilled Chicken

Difficulty Level: 2/5

Preparation time: 10 minutes

Cooking time: 20 minutes

Servings: 4

Ingredients:

½ c. lemon juice

½ c. extra-virgin olive oil

3 tbsps. minced garlic

2 tsps. dried oregano

1 tsp. red pepper flakes

1 tsp. salt

2 lbs. or 900 g boneless chicken breasts, skinless

Directions:

In a medium bowl, combine garlic, lemon juice, olive oil, oregano, red pepper flakes, and salt.

Divide chicken breast horizontally to get 2 thin pieces. Repeat this process with the rest chicken breasts.

Set the chicken in the bowl with the marinade and let sit for at least 10 minutes before cooking.

Place the skillet on a high heat and add oil.

Cook each side of the breasts for 4 minutes.

Serve warm.

Nutrition:

Calories 479

Fat 32 g

Sat fat 5 g

Fiber 1 g

Carbohydrates 5 g

Sugars 1 g

Protein 47 g

Sodium 943 mg

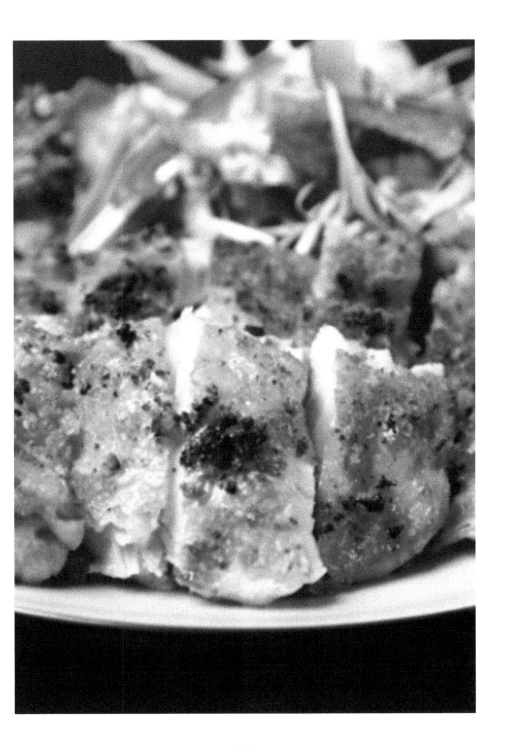

Pasta with Creamy Tomato Sauce

Difficulty Level: 3/5

Preparation time: 10 minutes

Cooking time: 10 minutes

Servings: 4

Ingredients:

16 ounces linguine

2 cups chopped onion

1 cup chopped carrot

½ cup dry white wine

½ cup raw unsalted cashew pieces

¼ to ½ cup of water

2 (14.5-ounce) cans diced tomatoes

4 garlic cloves, peeled

24 large basil leaves, 12 left whole and 12 cut into thin ribbons

1 teaspoon of sea salt

¼ teaspoon freshly ground black pepper

Directions:

Bring a large pot of water to a boil over high heat and cook the pasta until al dente according to the directions on the package. Drain.

Meanwhile, in a large skillet, combine the onion, carrot, and wine. (If you're not using a high-speed blender, add the cashews now as well.) Sauté the vegetables over medium heat for 5 minutes, stirring often. As you go, add the water, as needed, to prevent sticking.

.Add the tomatoes and their juices. Cook, often stirring, for another 5 minutes.

Transfer the mixture to a high-speed blender. Add the garlic, whole basil leaves, cashews, salt, and pepper. Blend until very smooth.

Serve generous portions of the sauce over the pasta and top with the fresh basil ribbons.

Nutrition:

Calories: 532;

Total Fat: 11g;

Saturated Fat: 2g;

Protein: 17g;

Carbohydrates: 85g;

Fiber: 8g;

Sodium: 503mg;

Iron: 4mg

Greek Tostadas

Difficulty Level: 2/5

Preparation time: 15 minutes

Cooking time: 10 minutes

Servings: 6

Ingredients:

Olive oil cooking spray

6 (6-inch) corn tortillas

7 cups stemmed and finely chopped lacinato or curly kale

2 tablespoons freshly squeezed lemon juice

1 tablespoon extra-virgin olive oil

2 garlic cloves, minced or pressed

¼ teaspoon of sea salt

1 recipe Happy Hummus

2 avocados, peeled, pitted, and chopped

¾ cup finely chopped purple cabbage

2 tomatoes, chopped

2 limes or lemons, quartered (optional)

Directions:

Preheat the oven to 400°F. Spray a rimmed baking sheet with cooking spray.

Arrange the tortillas in a single layer on the prepared sheet. Spray the tops generously with oil and bake for 5 to 10 minutes until lightly browned and crisp. Set aside.

In a large bowl, combine the kale, lemon juice, and olive oil. Using your hands, work the lemon and oil into the kale, squeezing firmly, so that the kale becomes soft and tenderized, as well as a darker shade of green. Stir in the garlic and salt.

To assemble, top the baked tortillas with a generous layer of hummus. Top evenly with the massaged kale, avocado chunks, cabbage, and tomatoes. If desired, serve with lime or lemon wedges for squeezing over the top.

Nutrition:

Calories: 474;

Total Fat: 28g;

Saturated Fat: 4g;

Protein: 13g;

Carbohydrates: 48g;

Fiber: 13g;

Sodium: 307mg;

Iron: 5mg

Chickpea Medley

Difficulty Level: 1/5

Preparation time: 5 minutes

Cooking time: 0 minutes

Servings: 2

Ingredients:

2 tablespoons tahini

2 tablespoons coconut aminos

1 (15-ounce) can chickpeas or 1½ cups cooked chickpeas, rinsed and drained

1 cup finely chopped lightly packed spinach

1 carrot, peeled and grated

Directions:

In a medium bowl, whisk together the tahini and coconut aminos.

Add the chickpeas, spinach, and carrot to the bowl. Stir well and serve at room temperature. Store leftovers in an airtight container in the refrigerator for up to 1 week.

Nutrition:

Calories: 161;

Total Fat: 6g;

Saturated Fat: 1g;

Protein: 7g;

Carbohydrates: 22g;

Fiber: 6g;

Sodium: 38mg;

Iron: 3mg

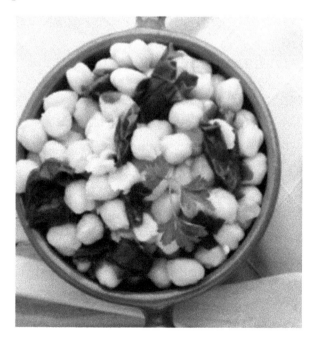

Moroccan Couscous

Difficulty Level: 2/5

Preparation time: 10 minutes

Cooking time: 5 minutes

Servings: 5

Ingredients:

1 cup couscous

1½ cups water

1½ teaspoons grated orange or lemon zest

¾ cup freshly squeezed orange juice

4 or 5 garlic cloves, minced or pressed

2 tablespoons raisins

2 tablespoons pure maple syrup or agave nectar

2¼ teaspoons ground cumin

2¼ teaspoons ground cinnamon

¼ teaspoon paprika

2½ tablespoons minced fresh mint

2 teaspoons freshly squeezed lemon juice

½ teaspoon of sea salt

Directions:

In a medium pot, combine the couscous and water. Add the orange zest and juice, garlic, raisins, maple syrup, cumin, cinnamon, and paprika and stir. Bring the mixture to a boil over medium-high heat.

Remove the couscous from the heat and stir well. Cover with a tight-fitting lid and set aside until all of the liquids are absorbed and the couscous is tender and fluffy. Gently stir in the mint, lemon juice, and salt. Serve warm or cold. Store leftovers in an airtight container in the refrigerator for up to 5 days.

Nutrition:

Calories: 242;

Total Fat: 1g;

Saturated Fat: 0g;

Protein: 7g;

Carbohydrates: 53g;

Fiber: 3g;

Sodium: 244mg;

Iron: 2mg

Lemony Asparagus Pasta

Difficulty Level: 2/5

Preparation time: 10 minutes

Cooking time: 20 minutes

Servings: 6

Ingredients:

1 pound spaghetti, linguini, or angel hair pasta

2 crusty bread slices

½ cup plus 1 tablespoon avocado oil, divided

3 cups chopped asparagus (1½-inch pieces)

½ cup vegan "chicken" broth or vegetable broth, divided

6 tablespoons freshly squeezed lemon juice

8 garlic cloves, minced or pressed

3 tablespoons finely chopped fresh curly parsley

1 tablespoon grated lemon zest

1½ teaspoons sea salt

Directions:

Bring a large pot of water to a boil over high heat and cook the pasta until al dente according to the instructions on the package.

Meanwhile, in a medium skillet, crumble the bread into coarse crumbs. Add 1 tablespoon of oil to the pan and stir well to combine over medium heat. Cook for about 5 minutes, stirring often, until the crumbs are golden brown. Remove from the skillet and set aside.

Add the chopped asparagus and ¼ cup of broth in the skillet and cook over medium-high heat until the asparagus is bright green and crisp-tender, about 5 minutes. Transfer the asparagus to a very large bowl.

Add the remaining ½ cup of oil, remaining ¼ cup of broth, lemon juice, garlic, parsley, zest, and salt to the asparagus bowl and stir well.

When the noodles are done, drain well, and add them to the bowl. Gently toss with the asparagus mixture. Just before serving, stir in the toasted bread crumbs. Store leftovers in an airtight container in the refrigerator for up 2 days.

Nutrition:

Calories: 526;

Total Fat: 23g;

Saturated Fat: 3g;

Protein: 13g;

Carbohydrates: 68g;

Fiber: 10g;

Sodium: 1422mg;

Iron: 6mg

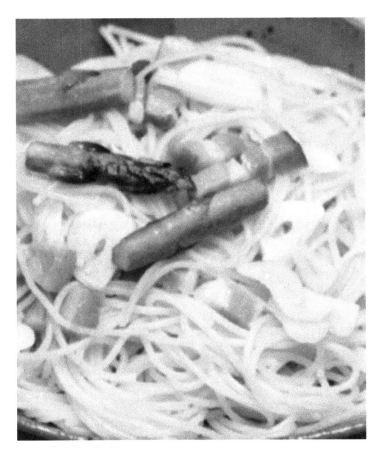

Mediterranean Grilled Shrimp

Difficulty Level: 2/5

Preparation time: 20 minutes

Cooking time: 5 minutes

Servings: 4-7

Ingredients:

2 tablespoons garlic, minced

½ cup lemon juice

3 tablespoons fresh Italian parsley, finely chopped

¼ cup extra-virgin olive oil

1 teaspoon salt

2 pounds jumbo shrimp (21-25), peeled and deveined

Directions:

In a large bowl, mix the garlic, lemon juice, parsley, olive oil, and salt.

Add the shrimp to the bowl and toss to make sure all the pieces are coated with the marinade. Let the shrimp sit for 15 minutes.

Preheat a grill, grill pan, or lightly oiled skillet to high heat. While heating, thread about 5 to 6 pieces of shrimp onto each skewer.

Place the skewers on the grill, grill pan, or skillet and cook for 2 to 3 minutes on each side until cooked through. Serve warm.

Nutrition:

Calories: 402;

Protein: 57g;

Total
Carbohydrates: 4g;

Sugars: 1g;

Fiber: 0g;

Total Fat: 18g;

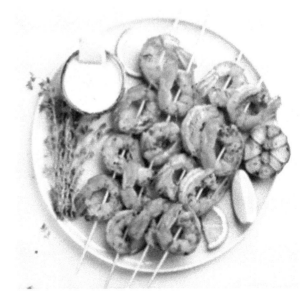

Italian Breaded Shrimp

Difficulty Level: 2/5

Preparation time: 10 minutes

Cooking time: 5 minutes

Servings: 4

Ingredients:

2 large eggs

2 cups seasoned Italian breadcrumbs

1 teaspoon salt

1 cup flour

1 pound large shrimp (21-25), peeled and deveined

Extra-virgin olive oil

Directions:

In a small bowl, beat the eggs with 1 tablespoon water, then transfer to a shallow dish.

Add the breadcrumbs and salt to a separate shallow dish; mix well.

Place the flour into a third shallow dish.

Coat the shrimp in the flour, then egg, and finally the breadcrumbs. Place on a plate and repeat with all of the shrimp.

Preheat a skillet over high heat. Pour in enough olive oil to coat the bottom of the skillet. Cook the shrimp in the hot skillet for 2 to 3 minutes on each side. Take the shrimp out and drain on a paper towel. Serve warm.

Nutrition:

Calories: 714;

Protein: 37g;

Total Carbohydrates: 63g;

Sugars: 4g;

Fiber: 3g;

Total Fat: 34g

Fried Fresh Sardines

Preparation time: 5 minutes

Cooking time: 5 minutes

Servings: 4

Ingredients:

Avocado oil

1½ pounds whole fresh sardines, scales removed

1 teaspoon salt

1 teaspoon freshly ground black pepper

2 cups flour

Directions:

Preheat a deep skillet over medium heat. Pour in enough oil so there is about 1 inch of it in the pan.

Season the fish with the salt and pepper.

Dredge the fish in the flour so it is completely covered.

Slowly drop in 1 fish at a time, making sure not to overcrowd the pan.

Cook for about 3 minutes on each side or just until the fish is golden brown on all sides. Serve warm.

Nutrition:

Calories: 794;

Protein: 48g;

Total Carbohydrates: 44g;

Fiber: 2g;

Total Fat: 47g

White Wine–Sautéed Mussels

Difficulty Level: 2/5

Preparation time: 10 minutes

Cooking time: 10 minutes

Servings: 4

Ingredients:

3 pounds live mussels, cleaned

4 tablespoons (½ stick) salted butter

2 shallots, finely chopped

2 tablespoons garlic, minced

2 cups dry white wine

Directions:

Scrub the mussel shells to make sure they are clean; trim off any that have a beard (hanging string). Put the mussels in a large bowl of water, discarding any that are not tightly closed.

In a large pot over medium heat, cook the butter, shallots, and garlic for 2 minutes.

Add the wine to the pot, and cook for 1 minute.

Add the mussels to the pot, toss with the sauce, and cover with a lid. Let cook for 7 minutes. Discard any mussels that have not opened.

Serve in bowls with the wine broth.

Nutrition:

Calories: 777;

Protein: 82g;

Total Carbohydrates: 29g;

Sugars: 1g;

Total Fat: 27g;

Saturated Fat: 10g

Chicken Shawarma

Difficulty Level: 2/5

Preparation time: 15 minutes

Cooking time: 15 minutes

Servings: 4

Ingredients:

2 pounds boneless and skinless chicken

½ cup lemon juice

½ cup extra-virgin olive oil

3 tablespoons minced garlic

1½ teaspoons salt

½ teaspoon freshly ground black pepper

½ teaspoon ground cardamom

½ teaspoon cinnamon

Hummus and pita bread, for serving (optional)

Directions:

Cut the chicken into ¼-inch strips and put them into a large bowl.

In a separate bowl, whisk together the lemon juice, olive oil, garlic, salt, pepper, cardamom, and cinnamon.

Pour the dressing over the chicken and stir to coat all of the chicken.

Let the chicken sit for about 10 minutes.

Heat a large pan over medium-high heat and cook the chicken pieces for 12 minutes, using tongs to turn the chicken over every few minutes.

Serve with hummus and pita bread, if desired.

Nutrition:

Calories: 477;

Protein: 47g;

Total Carbohydrates: 5g;

Sugars: 1g;

Fiber: 1g;

Total Fat: 32g

Paprika-Spiced Fish

Difficulty Level: 2/5

Preparation time: 5 minutes

Cooking time: 10 minutes

Servings: 4

Ingredients:

4 (5-ounce) sea bass fillets

½ teaspoon salt

1 tablespoon smoked paprika

3 tablespoons unsalted butter

Lemon wedges

Directions:

Season the fish on both sides with the salt. Repeat with the paprika.

Preheat a skillet over high heat. Melt the butter.

Once the butter is melted, add the fish and cook for 4 minutes on each side.

Once the fish is done, move to a serving dish and squeeze lemon over the top.

Nutrition:

Calories: 257;

Protein: 34;

Total Carbohydrates: 1g;

Fiber: 1g;

Total Fat: 13g

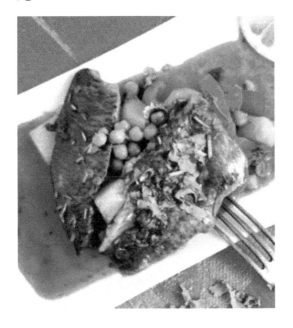

Greek Style Spring Soup

Difficulty Level: 2/5

Preparation Time: 10 minutes

Cooking time: 20 minutes

Servings: 4

Ingredients:

3 cups chicken stock

½ pound chicken breast, shredded

1 tablespoon chives, chopped

1 egg, whisked

½ white onion, diced

1 bell pepper, chopped

1 tablespoon olive oil

¼ cup Arborio rice

½ teaspoon salt

1 tablespoon fresh cilantro, chopped

Directions:

Pour olive oil in the stock pan and preheat it.

Add onion and bell pepper. Roast the vegetables for 3-4 minutes. Stir them from time to time.

After this, add rice and stir well.

Cook the ingredients for 3 minutes over the medium heat.

Then add chicken stock and stir the soup well.

Add salt and bring the soup to boil.

Add shredded chicken breast, cilantro, and chives. Add egg and stir it carefully.

Close the lid and simmer the soup for 5 minutes over the medium heat.

Remove the cooked soup from the heat.

Nutrition:

Calories 176

Fat 5.6 g

Fiber 7.6g

Carbohydrates 23.6 g

Protein 4.6 g

Avgolemono Soup

Difficulty Level: 2/5

Preparation Time: 10 minutes

Cooking time: 20 minutes

Servings: 6

Ingredients:

4 cups chicken stock

1 cup of water

1-pound chicken breast, shredded

1 cup of rice, cooked

3 egg yolks

3 tablespoons lemon juice

1/3 cup fresh parsley, chopped

½ teaspoon salt

¼ teaspoon ground black pepper

Directions:

Pour water and chicken stock in the saucepan and bring to boil.

Then pour one cup of the hot liquid in the food processor.

Add cooked rice, egg yolks, lemon juice, and salt. Blend the mixture until smooth.

After this, transfer the smooth rice mixture into the saucepan with remaining chicken stock liquid.

Add shredded chicken breast, parsley, and ground black pepper.

Boil the soup for 5 minutes more.

Nutrition:

Calories 235

Fat 5.6 g

Fiber 7.6g

Carbohydrates 23.6 g

Protein 4.6 g

Rosemary Minestrone

Difficulty Level: 2/5

Preparation Time: 5 minutes

Cooking time: 25 minutes

Servings: 4

Ingredients:

2 oz celery stalk, chopped

1 russet potato, chopped

½ cup butternut squash, chopped

1 teaspoon fresh rosemary

½ teaspoon salt

½ teaspoon ground black pepper

2 oz Parmesan, grated

1 tablespoon butter

½ zucchini, chopped

¼ cup green beans, chopped

2 oz whole wheat pasta

4 cups chicken stock

½ teaspoon tomato paste

¾ cup red kidney beans, canned, drained

Directions:

In the saucepan combine together celery stalk, potato, butternut squash, rosemary, salt, ground black pepper, butter, and stir well.

Cook the vegetables for 5 minutes over the medium-low heat.

After this, add zucchini, green beans, whole-wheat pasta, chicken stock, and tomato paste.

Add red kidney beans and chicken stock.

Stir the soup well and cook it for 15 minutes over the medium-high heat.

Then add Parmesan and stir minestrone.

Cook it for 2 minutes more.

Ladle minestrone in the serving bowls immediately.

Nutrition:

Calories 234

Fat 6.5

Fiber 10.1

Carbohydrates 39.7

Protein 31.1

Orzo Soup with Kale

Difficulty Level: 2/5

Preparation Time: 10 minutes

Cooking time: 20 minutes

Servings: 4

Ingredients:

1/3 cup orzo pasta

¼ white onion, diced

1 oz celery stalk, chopped

½ teaspoon chili flakes

½ teaspoon salt

1 garlic clove, diced

1 cup kale, chopped

½ cup tomatoes, chopped

1 carrot, chopped

½ teaspoon dried thyme

½ teaspoon dried oregano

5 cups vegetable stock

Directions:

Pour the vegetable stock in the pan and bring it to boil.

Add celery stalk and diced onion.

After this, sprinkle the liquid with chili flakes and salt.

Add diced garlic, tomatoes, carrot, dried thyme, and dried oregano.

Bring the liquid to boil.

Add orzo pasta and cook it for 5 minutes.

After this, add kale and cook the soup for 3 minutes more.

Remove the soup from the heat and leave it to rest with the closed lid for 10 minutes.

Nutrition:

Calories 74

Fat 6.5

Fiber 5.1

Carbohydrates 2.7

Braised Swiss Chard with Potatoes

Difficulty Level: 2/5

Preparation time: 5 minutes

Cooking time: 5 minutes

Serving: 4

Ingredients:

1 pound Swiss chard, torn, chopped with stems

2 potatoes, peeled and chopped

¼ tablespoon oregano

1 teaspoon salt

Directions:

Take a pot and add Swiss chard and potatoes to the pot

Pour water to cover all and sprinkle with salt

Close the lid and then press the Pressure cook/Manual button

Cook for 3 minutes on High

Release the steam naturally over 5 minutes

Sprinkle with Italian seasoning or oregano on top

Serve and enjoy!

Nutrition: (Per Serving)

Calories: 246

Fat: 10g

Carbohydrates: 29g

Protein: 12g

Mushroom and Vegetable Penne Pasta

Difficulty Level: 2/5

Preparation Time: 5 minutes

Cooking Time: 8 minutes

Serving: 4

Ingredients:

6 ounces penne pasta

6 ounces shitake mushrooms, chopped

1 small carrot, cut into strips

4 ounces baby spinach, finely chopped

1 teaspoon ginger, grounded

3 tablespoons oil

2 tablespoons soy sauce

6 ounces zucchini, cut into strips

6 ounces leek, finely chopped

½ teaspoon salt

2 garlic cloves, crushed

2 cups of water

Directions:

Heat the oil

Sauté and stir-fry carrot and garlic for 3-4 minutes

Add remaining ingredients and pour in 2 cups water

Cook on High pressure for 4 minutes

Quick-release the pressure

Serve and enjoy!

Nutrition: (Per Serving)

Calories: 429

Fat: 8g

Carbohydrates: 64g

Protein: 25g

Mushroom Spinach Tagliatelle

Difficulty Level: 2/5

Preparation time: 10 minutes

Cooking time: 5 minutes

Serving: 4

Ingredients:

1 pound tagliatelle

¼ cup parmesan cheese, grated

2 garlic cloves, crushed

¼ cup heavy cream

6 ounces mixed mushrooms, frozen

3 tablespoons coconut oil, unsalted

¼ cup feta cheese

1 tablespoon Italian seasoning mix

Directions:

Melt coconut oil on sauté

Stir-fry the garlic for a minute

Stir in feta and mushrooms

Add tagliatelle and 2 cups of water

Cook for 4 minutes on High pressure

Quick-release the pressure

Top with the parmesan

Serve and enjoy!

Nutrition: (Per Serving)

Calories: 298

Fat: 13g

Carbohydrates: 28g

Protein: 14g

Lightning Source UK Ltd.
Milton Keynes UK
UKHW020810110621
385331UK00004B/171